God's Health Care System

God Has His Own System That Works

Receiving Healing
Health Stories From
The Holy Bible

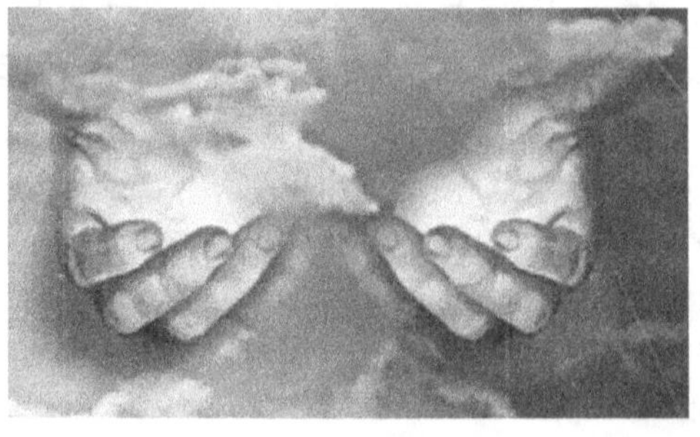

Book By

Shelly Jenkins, BSN, RN

God's Health Care System

God Has His Own System That Works

Receiving Healing Health Stories From

The Holy Bible

Copyright © 2017 Shelly Jenkins

ISBN-13:978-1983454899

ISBN-10:1983454893

Published by Kingdom Consulting and Publishing

Table of Contents

DEDICATION

To all who seek affirmation
that they have value.

Preface

Got unsolved problems, that is, got issues? Things that bother us or just aren't going the way we planned or hoped? Things we can't resolve? Many or should I more accurately say **all** of us do.

So what we need are answers and solutions to these problems. But we hear all the time that people have problems. We are hearing more and more about them publicly until it has become fashionable to tell everybody your problems. We get "too much information" from TV shows, "reality" talk shows, documentaries, and of course, the news media reporting them daily. It's the thing to thrive on now, the negativity. It's not the news that's news, it's the negativity that's news now. You can't even talk to someone now without an update on how bad it is. We snapshot it from our phones to Facebook or Tweet it on social media rapidly so that "the grapevine" is comparable to snail mail. I think the term is "going viral". Viral, that used to be something bad and now it's the goal of communications.

Now I don't say this because I lack compassion. I have to look at these things because they **are** a terrible testimony of how the world is getting worse and people are falling prey to its powers. But this is nothing new. For generations, this is the human plight.

As I read the story of a woman in the bible who was sick (chapter one), I thought "nothing has changed". This could easily be a twenty-first century woman having the same problems and still getting the same results, 2000 years later. It's remarkable to me that even with the advancements and resources we have at our finger tips, we are still getting the same results. People having problems for YEARS and no solution in sight.

Unable to get the answers they so desperately need (even in an information age). What are we doing wrong?

But God has a health care system (as I have explained in my previous books). Yes, His own system to take care of our health, and it works. It is different from the system that everybody commonly uses. The question is are you using it, or even aware of it? He has never intended for you to have the kind of problems that the earth cursed system produces. He does not want to leave you hanging in the balance of poor health. He knows what your needs are. Yes, in the twenty-first century we can get the results that the woman with the "issue" of blood did back then when she gave up on that system and turned to God's Health Care System.

Thank God some things don't change...

Chapter 1
What's Your Issue?

And a woman was there who had been subject to bleeding for twelve years. She had suffered a great deal under the care of many doctors and had spent all she had, yet instead of getting better she grew worse. When she heard about Jesus, she came up behind him in the crowd and touched his cloak, because she thought, "If I just touch his clothes, I will be healed." Immediately her bleeding stopped and she felt in her body that she was freed from her suffering.

At once Jesus realized that power had gone out from him. He turned around in the crowd and asked, "Who touched my clothes?"

"You see the people crowding against you," his disciples answered, "and yet you can ask, 'Who touched me?'"

But Jesus kept looking around to see who had done it. Then the woman, knowing what had happened to her, came and fell at his feet and, trembling with fear, told him the whole truth. He said to her, "Daughter, your faith has healed you. Go in peace and be freed from your suffering."   Mark 5: 25-34 (NLT)

Here is a woman with an issue of blood who suffered for 12 years! That's like prison time. And for her it was. Practically solitary confinement because she was considered "unclean" in her culture. This meant she was restricted in her contact with others. Isolated, you know, walled off from the flock (and you know what that means). It's the worst place you can be.

This was a woman who was using the earth cursed system of health (vs. God's Health Care System), and **could not get better**. Remember it says she suffered **12 years**, isolated and being socially unclean, abandoned by society. She thought "If I just touch his clothes (the hem), I will be healed" not him, just his garment...**the hem**. She touched his garment, a point of contact, as an **act of faith**. Healed!What a strategy!

I have to pause and think about her strategy because it seems insignificant... but it's not. And this is where we have to tweek our brains when using God's Health Care System. See, we think it takes a big deal to get healing so we don't demand it and we settle for less. But why not the **real** healing? Instead it's give me the hip replacement instead of the healed joint from supplements (especially, if you don't know there is a better way). We go for the elaborate, the $70,000 hysterectomy instead of a prayer of faith. We're trained to think it should be a big deal. But why not a simple act of faith by touching the hem of the Doctor's garment (The Great Physician), without the appointment, insurance and copay, just catching him walking down the proverbial street. It's too easy.

You can have an issue for a long time. Years before you finally recognize or realize that something is not working. That all this chaos you're going through is too much. And some of us never get there.

I used to pride myself on watching other people, you know people who are stuck and watch how their own situations played out. Then I would think to myself, "I don't want that to happen to me". I would take their hard won experience and not make the same mistake. I would consider it a blessing that I didn't have to go throught all that to find out what they had learned.

I had a girlfriend once, she was crazy about this guy. He was attractive and seemed like a strong young man. He eventually became unfaithful and left her for another woman. But not before she slept with him and became pregnant. She opted to not keep her baby. She was so sad that he left her alone even knowing her situation. Many years later, guess who shows up again? Yep, him. Guess what happened? She trusted him again and they started dating. Then guess what happened? Yep, she got pregnant again. **And then** guess what happened? Yep, he left her twice. And furthermore, guess what she did in her now complete despair? She did what she did with her first baby. It was hard to support her through that and watch her heart get broken not once but **twice**. But you think I didn't learn something from that? Think again!

First, I learned that some things don't change. I believe once a track record is set, it's set. It won't change. Do people change? It's possible I guess, but

I learned that you better have some sort of system in place to help you determine what risks you are willing to take and which ones are NOT worth it.

For me, I give you a chance the first time but usually not the second. I'd rather give that second chance to someone new but not the same person again. What do they say, "first time shame on you, second time, shame on me."

Let's break this down. The issue was bleeding. The Greek term used here is stanch, meaning to stop or restrict a flow of blood like from a wound.

So she had **a wound** that wouldn't heal and kept bleeding, which could be secondary to a more grave condition.

"...and had suffered a great deal under the care of many doctors..."

Okay, sorry guys but I'm going to get started here. It's incredible to me to think that I could make some **small sacrifices** that would pay **great dividends** when it comes to my health. I have talked to two men in two weeks recently who would not even entertain a discussion on lifestyle changes (small sacrifices). One is already

on meds for a serious condition
and another who has suffered 3
serious incidents and the
subsequent hospitalizations for a
life-threatening condition. It's
no wonder the physicians say,
"Just take their money", it's a no
brainer. I can get rich because
you'll never change. Wow!

Now lifestyle changes, in
many cases, can take great
efforts. But most times, they
really don't. And in most cases,
one can't do it alone. But how
bad does it have to get to take
some gentle suggestions or
some "FREE" advice.

I usually get stonewalled trying to reason with patients. I realize people do not recognize what the real cost or the consequences of their lifestyles are. Then they try to get well. They may believe that things will get better, BUT THEY DON'T. They spend more effort getting worse than they do getting better (you should read that again).

Now, I do realize the state that people are in from the earth cursed system of health. Once you start to make the changes, you don't see light at the end of the tunnel immediately. But if you give it some time, the results are quite miraculous. Then you can't stop going now because you're too geeked. Now you got a result that most people won't believe, others would "die for" and everybody will definitely be jealous of.

I love it when I tell people that I can feel that my knee joints aren't just pain free now but that the joint seems as if it has been reconstructed. This is just from abstaining from wheat and taking a bone-restoring supplement for about a month and a half now. The joint feels stronger. When I first stopped eating wheat (which incidentally cured my arthritis), I didn't miss it because I was too busy waiting for the results I had heard about from a friend. Now I can do child's posture in Yoga class without pain and with more flexibility. This is a big difference in my knees from when I was taking steroid injections just so I could walk. They told me the injections would not work forever. I was heading for knee replacement twice in a life time because I was still relatively young (in my forties). They'd have to replace the replacement in 10 years.

"and had spent all she had, yet instead of getting better she grew worse."

Oh how her finances would improve, and greatly at that! She would no longer have to search for or travel to "the next doctor" to see if he could cure her. No more going through medication trials or therapeutic procedures (I'm sure they had them back then). No disappointment from failed attempts that work on your self-esteem because you "made another bad decision". No more suffering because she was weak and could not take care of herself while she was bleeding to death. No more changing clothes constantly or ruining them. No more social isolations. She could now go wherever she wanted to and have meaningful new opportunites and relationships! That constitutes emotional recovery. Wow!

"When she heard about Jesus, she came up behind him through the crowd and touched his robe. For she thought to herself, "If I can just touch his robe, I will be healed."

Here is when you get so desperate that you're through making appointments where you just have to be squeezed in. So desperate that you need help quick and in a hurry and you won't be fooled anymore that something else was going to help you.

She caught Jesus on his way to "another appointment", as he was going to Jairus' house to heal his daughter. Jairus, mind you, was a leader of the local synagogue. No doubt a person of some standing in the community. Someone who could get "an appointment" just because he was *that* person. And Jairus had a more serious problem than she had. His daughter was dying (you know, the sign on the ER wall that states "WE SEE THE MOST SERIOUS PERSON FIRST"). The sign that could bump you down the waiting list for a few hours, right?

But funny, with God's health care system she didn't get bumped down, nor did she have to wait because she realized that if she could just "touch the hem of his garment" (a God revelation), she would be healed. I get peace just hearing how that sounds and thinking about how easy it is. So she did, and it made her an instant appointment!

"Jesus realized at once that power had gone out from him, so he turned around in the crowd and asked, "Who touched my robe?"

His disciples said to him, "Look at this crowd pressing around you. How can you ask, 'Who touched me?'"

Jesus knew immediately that something had happened.

He stops and says, "Who touched me?" She got bumped up the schedule to see the real doctor. Would your doctor do that yet alone make a home visit (like Jairus was getting ready to get)? Have you asked for a God revelation about your health issue lately? Did you recognize that this doctor was easily accessible? Walking around the community, not in that downtown office or medical campus office. It's so congested in those places, you know, the parking and all.

I stop here because I am amazed that Jesus in such a large crowd could perceive that power had gone out of him. Was he able to feel the demands of so many people and their needs as it states here? But I realized no, not everyone, just those with faith in the kingdom and its ability to heal them. Just those able to tap into the power and draw from it.

And furthermore, I am awestruck at his response to so little an act by an unknown person. He begins to make this big deal out of one person, in a crowd, while on his way to an emergency situation! He made the time for it and insisted on knowing! Why? I think it is because Jesus was always looking for someone who was getting the message of what His health care system, the kingdom of God, is all about. They are people he wants to praise and say, "see look at this person, they know how my kingdom is operating". No "O ye of little faith" here.

But then his disciples who **not** knowing the significance of what had happened stated in essence, "all these people here, so what?" But he continues to insist, or make a big stink, lol and says "who touched my garment!"

"But He kept looking around to see who had done it. Then the frightened woman, trembling at the realization of what had happened to her, came and fell to her knees in front of

him and, told him what she had done."

And with the desire to meet this person who had drawn out this power from the kingdom, he turns. Then the woman who knows that you **don't have to talk to him, just turn to him** was being called out. Something she didn't intend to happen. She was so used to being ignored and abandoned that she didn't think that her strategy, her approach or method to get what she needed would change her usual treatment. But not so, the master's response was quite different. And I think deep in her heart she was hoping that the results she got from Jesus would be different. And they were, for she knew in that instance that she had gotten healing in her body. She was now afraid of probably being chastised for taking that power from him when in all actuality this is exactly what God wants us to do. Take what belongs to us, because it's our inheritance. So much so that he wanted to publicly acknowledge her faith in His health care system, publicly acknowledge her, publicly acknowledge the kingdom, and publicly acknowledge His purpose for being here. He affirms her healing as a doctor would confirm that your cancer is gone, or your test results are negative.

"He said to her, "Daughter,"
I also believe that God wants to make her an example too of how important we are to Him. Of the value and worth we have to Him because next he responds by this remark:

"Daughter (of the kingdom), your faith has made you well." He calls her daughter, a member of the family, and tells her why he is praising her act. It was her faith or right standing **by actions** that got her needs met. Many of us do not realize that our right action is what proves that we are children of God.

"your faith has made you well."

With God it's not humiliation but affirmation. Our affirmations "If I could but touch the hem of his garment,"can build our faith up. However, it alone will not heal us even though we must speak in order to exercise our authority. Our faith without action will not heal us. The action connects us to the power.

He says to her, your faith has made you well because he wants us to know we have the power to choose our destiny regarding healing, our infirmity does not have to make that choice for us. No disease should ever have bullying rights.

"Go in peace"

Why was it important to say that? Because how often do we ignore that when our health is not good, it wears away our peace of mind. We worry about whether we will get better. Scheming about how we will try to get that office near the bathroom because of our infirmity. Or planning our day around public transportation services for the handicap to get to that doctor visit. Or waiting on hold for 30 minutes to talk to billing, or to get that appointment, or talk to the health care worker.

Peace of mind is a great commodity. Jesus mentioned to the woman to "Go in Peace" because he knew the significance and freedom she would have to **get on** with her life now that she would **not** have to be preoccupied with medical issues. Freedom, something she could now celebrate in.

"and be freed from your suffering."

Your verdict will always be wholeness. A complete healing; mind, body and soul, from your plague or your "disastrous evil affliction" or calamity. Yes, everything that is connected to this problem. It's now disconnected. It's over, amen.

Chapter 2
Well Watching

Ever felt destitute
(meaning lacking something
needed or desirable; lack of
resources, suffering extreme
poverty)? This story (John 4: 4-
38), is not so much about
physical healings, as many of the
stories in this book, as it is about
the emotional or soul healings
that God wants to address in our
lives. Remember, He isn't giving
this information to us without a
purpose or strategy for us to
embrace. Read this story:

Eventually he came to the Samaritan village of Sychar, near the field that Jacob gave to his son Joseph. Jacob's well was there; and Jesus, tired from the long walk, sat wearily beside the well about noontime. Soon a Samaritan woman came to draw water, and Jesus said to her, "Please give me a drink." He was alone at the time because his disciples had gone into the village to buy some food.

The woman was surprised, for Jews refuse to have anything to do with Samaritans. She said to Jesus, "You are a Jew, and I am a Samaritan woman. Why

are you asking me for a drink?
Jesus replied, "If you only knew
the gift God has for you and who
you are speaking to, you would
ask me, and I would give you
living water."

    "But sir, you don't have a
rope or a bucket," she said, "and
this well is very deep. Where
would you get this livin water?
And besides, do you think you're
greater than our ancestor Jacob,
who gave us this well? How can
you offer better water than he
and his sons and his animals
enjoyed?"

    Jesus replied, "Anyone who
drinks this water will soon

become thisty again. But those who drink the water I give will never be thirst again. It becomes a fresh, bubbling spring within them, giving them eternal life."

"Please, sir, " the woman said, "give me this water! Then I'll never be thirsty again, and I won't have to come here to get water."

"Go and get your husband." Jesus told her. "I don't have a husband," the woman replied.

Jesus said, "You're right! You don't have a husband – for you have had five husgands, and you aren't even married to the

man you're living with now. You
certainly spoke the truth!"

"Sir," the woman said, "you
must be a prophet. So tell me,
why is it that you Jews say that
Jerusalem is the only place of
worshp, while we Samaritans
claim it is here a Mount Gerzim,
where our ancestors
worshiped?"

Jesus replied, *"Believe me,
dear woman, the time is coming
when it will no longer matter
whether you worship the Father
on this mountain or in Jerusalem.
You Samaritans know very little
about the one you worship, while
we Jews know all about him for*

salvation comes through the Jews. But the time is coming indeed it's here now when true worshipers will worship he Father in pirit and in truth. The Father is looking for those who will worship him that way. For God is Spirit, so those who worship him must worship in spirit and in truth."

The woman said, "I know the Messiah is coming — the one who is called Christ. When he comes, he will explain everthing to us. Then Jesus told her, *"I AM the Messiah!"*

Just then his disciples came back. They were shocked to find *him talking to a woman, but non of had the nerve to ask, "What do you want with her?" or "Why are you talking to her?" The woman left her water jar beside the well and ran back to the village, telling everyone, "Come and see a man who told me everything I ever did! Could he possibly be the Messiah? So the people came streaming from the village to see him.*

Many Smaritans from the village believed in Jesus because the woman had said, "He told me everything I ever did! When they came out to see him, they begged him to stay in their village. So he stayed for two days, long enough for many more to hear his message and believe. Then they said to the woman, "Now we believe, not just because of what you told us, but because we have heard him ourselves. Now we know that he is indeed the Savior of the World."

John 4:4-33, 39-42 (NLT)

This story addresses, I believe, a woman with addictions. Addictions are the things we try, to get our needs met in the wrong way. Doing the same things over and over again, expecting different results. Until yep, we're stuck and we don't know it. We get caught in binging cycles (not just with food), and we can't get out. It is strange that this woman who had lived for carnal pleasures with men should feel this way, for she had not thought too much about her soul. Many women like this also have alcohol problems too, thus "give me a drink" would sound so familiar to her.

So a woman comes to the well for water and meets Jesus as he is siting there resting. Watching, no doubt, what people do when they come to a central place that is essential for meeting a life need, a well, to meet the need for water. A place where people come to satisfy **thirst**. But he knows its not just physical thirst people have, but emotional and spiritual thirst. The need we are unaware of or forget about or "dumb down" its significance. She is a woman from Samaria, and Jews don't even talk to them. But Jesus, a Jew, asks her for a drink of water. Water is so important to us physically, but here Jesus'conversation is regarding the spiritual. Yes, our spiritual need is God's first concern. Why? Because he knows the enemy wants to take us out before we get a handle on it and then it will be too late to do anything about it. Our fate is sealed. This is the health we don't covet like we do our physical health, it goes neglected even though it is the part of us that is eternal.

He let's her know that today is her day, in so many words because he has a gift for her, **living water**. Water that doesn't run out, that changes your life and your direction. For her, this encounter meant the

end of being stuck, the turning
point, the answer. He
prophetically tells her he knows
what's going on in her life (living
with numerous men...5
husbands and working on
number 6), but he doesn't
condemn her. He tells her that
now she will never have to go
from relationship to relationship,
thirsting, but that now she will
have a well, ON THE INSIDE OF
HER (where the hole can be
pretty big), a fresh bubbling
spring of water within her that
will bring her the eternal life,
(what she will really need and is
really searching for), but could

not find in men. Water for today and forever. Remember Jesus said in the Beattitudes,

"Blessed are those who do hunger and thirst after righteousness (or justice) they will be filled (or satisfied).

Matthew 5:6 (NKJ)

I noticed that when Jesus responded to her, he stepped over the race issue and went immediately to the kingdom **mindset** stating that God had a gift for her. She responds in a mindset of the issues and things of this life and how we get bogged down in the cares of life.

She did not realize that someone had a gift to give to her. He even gave away the answer to the test question by telling her how to get the gift that she doesn't even pick up on. Then he even tells her what the gift is. But she continues to tell him what he doesn't have, in other words, what is hindering **him** (sound familiar). Then becomes proud minded by saying your living water can't compare to our water from "Jacob's well". Jesus, knowing the culture knew that even a famous well will not get you the answers you seek in life. Kinda like name brand shoes, it's not **true** riches.

Many people go to the earth cursed system for therapy to help them figure out what's going wrong in their life. But how many will tell you that you need living water so you don't thirst any more. Or how many therapist will tell you that your problems are spiritual emptiness and emotional hunger. With most addictions, it is said if you want to know what's eating you, stop eating and you'll find out. Once an addict abstains, the reason he uses his addiction will become clear. Jesus told the woman that her solution was something, a gift that only comes from God. Which means that the gift had to be spiritual in nature. That is something you can't get from, health care professional or the earth cursed system.

Chapter 3
Give it to the Dog

"Then Jesus left Galilee and went north to the region of Tyre. He didn't want anyone to know which house he was staying in, but he couldn't keep it a secret. Right away a woman who had heard about him came and fell at his feet. Her little girl was possessed by an evil spirit, and she begged him to cast out the demon from her daughter.

Since she was a Gentile, born in Syrian Phoenicia, Jesus told her, "First I should feed the children—my own family, the

Jews. It isn't right to take food from the children and throw it to the dogs."

She replied, "That's true, Lord, but even the dogs under the table are allowed to eat the scraps from the children's plates."

"Good answer!" **He said.** *"Now go home, for the demon has left your daughter."* **And when she arrived home, she found her little girl lying quietly in bed, and the demon was gone.**
Mark 7:24-30 (NLT)

Humility and wisdom are elements that are discovered in this incident with yet another desparate woman who has an emotional problem with her teenager. How many of us know a parent who has trouble with their teenage kids. And the toughest problems with kids are emotional.

I worked in a school full of kids that had emotional problems. On the first day I was sent there, I got called to the office to meet a grandparent who was raising two boys with emotional problems. When I walked into the office, one of the them was on the floor screaming as if demon possessed. I immediately felt like this new assignment was a big mistake. I know that I stood there with a shocked look on my face before I could pull myself together. I had no skills whatsoever to deal with the situation and was unfamiliar with this student.

There has got to be people out there who know what this is like and are in the same situations. So you can see why this woman fell at Jesus feet and begged him to help her, as if this was the last straw.

God didn't leave her hanging. Even though he quoted the usual procedure to her to validate what his true mission was; feed the family of the Jewish Nation, he was humble enough to listen to her desparate cry for help. Her response was one he did not expect. Especially, considering the fact that his response would have offended the average person by implying that she was catagorized with the "dogs" of life. Wow, that could have stopped a person in their tracks you would think. But it didn't because she told him she at least deserved what was left, the crumbs.

The gospel of Matthew in the King James version says it this way:

"Truth, Lord: yet the dogs eat of the crumbs which fall from their masters' table.."

Matthew 15:27 (KJV)

She wanted him to remove the racial/religious problem (her ethnicity, being a Gentile) to get to the healing problem. She didn't get offended but said metaphorically that in my humanity there has got to be something for me.

In God's Health Care System, you get a piece of the pie, always. With God little, (the crumbs), is much. I remember alter calls as a child where they tell people "there's room at the alter for you". I love that all inclusive system of God. Just like the sun that shines down on everyone, whether you're a good or bad person. The compassion of God in his health care system is a continual theme in the healing arena.

Most importantly we know this mom had no other way to have her teen cured. And she didn't even bring her to Jesus. It could be that she was to emotionally ill to bring her daughter to Jesus and had to

seek him out. I noticed that
Jesus sent his power to those
who could not come to him if
others interceded for them.
Another action that you won't
see in the earth curse system!

Chapter 4

You Give Me Fever

"Jesus leaving the synagogue that day, went to Simon's home, where he found Simon's mother-in-law very sick with a high fever. "Please heal her," everyone begged. Standing at her bedside, he rebuked the fever, and it left her. And she got up at once and prepared a meal for them."

Luke 4: 38-39 (NLT)

Jesus heals the mother of Simon,who later was given a

new name and became his head disciple Peter. He had the true revelation of who Jesus really was after seeing all the wisdom and miracles Jesus had performed. He was the only disciple who was convinced that Jesus was not merely another prophet or teacher. Others told Jesus of his mother's problem (intercessory prayer) and he immediately addressed her sickness.

It wasn't just a fever but a "high" fever. Luke, who was also a physician and writer of this gospel, specifically uses the word "megas" in the greek manuscript. Fevers affects the blood pH. PH level are very precise which means there is a very small range for normal function. Proper pH ensures the uptake of minerals (we use 60 of them in our bodies), which are vital to our survival. The importance of proper pH function in our bodies is known by God. It is his wish for us to have these problems restored to its proper balance and range.

Mark states that Jesus not only healed her of the fever but he helped her "sit up" to assist her to a position where she could function again. He doesn't leave us in positions where we cannot function. Psalms 18 and 113 gently states the he "lifts me up" eluding to our physical, emotional and spiritual states.

The book of Matthew states:

"he touched her hand and she arose, and ministered unto them".

Matthew 8:14 (KJV)

I think the small phrase used here has meaning because she immediately was healed and begain to used her hands to serve him. In the kingdom, the point of touch is as important as the healing itself because it points to spiritual ramifications of our call and purpose. If we especially need a particular part of our body for kingdom service, God will use this area as a direct entry of His power to release you for service.

Chapter 5
HOLIDAYS!

The Crooked Woman of 18 Years

"One Sabbath day as Jesus was teaching in a synagogue, he saw a woman who had been crippled by an evil spirit. She had been bent double for eighteen years and was unable to stand up straight. When Jesus saw her, he called her over and said, "Dear woman, you are healed of your sickness!" Then he touched her, and instantly she could stand straight. How she praised God! But the leader in charge of

the synagogue was indignant
that Jesus had healed her on the
Sabbath day. "There are six days
of the week for working," he said
to the crowd. "Come on those
days to be healed, not on the
Sabbath." But the Lord replied,
"You hypocrites! Each of you
works on the Sabbath day! Don't
you untie your ox or your donkey
from its stall on the Sabbath and
lead it out for water? This dear
woman, a daughter of Abraham,
has been held in bondage by
Satan for eighteen years. Isn't it
right that she be released even
on the Sabbath?" This shamed
his enemies, but all the people

How long do we have to suffer? Can it be compared to anything else. Can it be measured, like a price on a piece of merchandise? Like tears, how much are they worth? It amazes me that the legal field like to compensate you for your "pain and suffering". How do they calculate that? How can you calculate the physical, emotional and spiritual effects of my illness. It effects generations. I think that the longer the condition exists, the amount of pain and suffering multiplies. That's the "design of devastion". It's why you can't get out on your own.

The term used in this passage for the infirmity "bent over double" is the greek word "sugkuptousa" meaning a curvature of the spine. In modern day venacular it is kyphotic spine or hunch back. Furthermore, Jesus, the Great Physician, gives the cause of the problem, a demonic infirmity (astheneias in greek) and speaks to it accurately by saying "thou art loosed.(KJV)" The greek medical term used here by the writer Luke is "apolelusai" referring to the relaxing of tendons or tight skin, or even removing bandages. This condition actually occurs from a large tendon in the back area that pulls the upper spine downward as it gradually contracts causing pain and difficulty breathing because the lungs can't expand.

So here Jesus rescues a "dear woman" and pronounces her verdict, "You are healed of your sickness", and pounds his gavel! Then with his personal attention, touches her and instantly she could stand straight!

He wouldn't let her stay that way. I love a God that won't let you "stay that way". He recognizes the abbnormal and demands that it be made right. When he saw her condition, he immediately dealt with it. No elephant in the living room. We can learn a lot from God. That's why he called her dear woman, she had value to Him. This is an important concept in the God's Health Care System. Your healing is based on your value. A single lost sheep, or one sparrow, a blade of grass, the hairs of your head being numbered, a plan for your life made even before the foundations of the earth.

But let's not forget her response…."How she praised God!" Or the crowds response. I think it got noisy up in there, right? Sports fans don't have nothing on a miracle healing. Better than a big lottery win! Your ship is coming in…this is your special day.

THE MAN WHO WAS SWOLLEN

"One Sabbath day Jesus went to eat dinner in the home

of a leader of the Pharisees, and the people were watching him closely. *There was a man there whose arms and legs were swollen* (congestive heart failure maybe, high blood pressure, kidneys failing?). *Jesus asked the Pharisees and experts in religious law, "Is it permitted in the law to heal people on the Sabbath day, or not?" When they refused to answer, Jesus touched the sick man and healed him and sent him away. Then he turned to them and said, "Which of you doesn't work on the Sabbath? If your son or cow (or donkey) falls into a pit, don't you rush to get him out?" Again they could not answer."*

Luke 14:1-6 (NLT)

Test time! Jesus posses a question, sort of a "pop quiz" asking them about Jewish etiquette. Funny how when we don't study regularly or are not "ready to give an answer on any occasion", we can't even make an intelligent guess. We just can't answer. So he asks what is the "religious"procedure? What rules are they living by? Ask yourself; have I ever been too confused about something I couldn't think of an answer? Or stubborn? Because it said they "refused" to answer. But remember there were supposed to be leaders among them (Pharisees and EXPERTS IN THE LAW) and THEY didn't answer the question either. Don't think for a minute that the proud among them didn't have an opinion or even knew the answer but no one was willing to state it because they were missing the spirit of the matter (that the Sabbath was created for man, not man for the Sabbath). That the event of healing allows us Sabbath rest or IS our Sabbath. No one was willing to go against the trend

that was being taught in *that* day
to give the answer to the
question. These are serious
heart issues because our healing
is at stake. What we are willing
to stand up for or support is
what we get in the kingdom. It's
not hard to get healed.

Jesus then, having more
desire to be compassionate than
politically correct, reaches over
to meet the need of the
individual man (before the public
opinion) and healed him right
before their eyes. Now if that
doesn't soften your heart, I don't
know what will. Then he did
more, he removed the man from

those who did not want what the kingdom had to offer, he sent him away! In other words, get away from these people so you can live a healed life! They will teach you and train you wrongly. They will keep you in unbelief. You could loose your soul.

THE MAN WITH THE DEFORMED HAND

On another Sabbath day, a man with a deformed right hand was in the synagogue while Jesus was teaching. The teachers of religious law and the Pharisees watched Jesus closely. If he healed the man's hand, they planned to accuse him of working on the Sabbath. "But Jesus knew their thoughts. He said to the man with the deformed hand, "Come and stand in front of everyone." So the man came forward. Then Jesus said to his critics, "I have a question for you. Does the law permit good deeds on the Sabbath, or is it a day for doing evil? Is this a day to save life or to destroy it?"

He looked around at them one by one and then said to the man, "Hold out your hand." So the man held out his hand, and it was restored! At this the *enemies of Jesus were wild with rage, and began to discuss what to do with him.*

Luke 6:6-11 (NLT)

Here was a man who came to the synagogue one day. I wonder if he ever thought when he got up that morning that when he came back home, he would have his hand restored. Jesus called him out as if to say "this is your day" but in a response to leaders who did not see the significance in meeting people's needs as paramount as keeping their religious traditions.

But Jesus uses this opportunity to impact this man's life and to show everyone that the intention of God is to make us whole. He asks the man to move openly in front of the people and asks the question that will help the people and the leaders understand how the kingdom of God or God's Health Care System works. A person in that society was probably pitied for so long and didn't feel very significant. But now he is standing before everyone with a healed hand. Now he has something new, freedom from pity and uniqueness. He is now blessed and better off than they are.

I would imagine that many were probably even mad that they couldn't work on the Sabbath (you know, to get ahead, like we do overtime to make up for our financial debts or deficits). Or they were being legalistic or "picking nits" since they were accusing Jesus of doing work. Even though for Jesus, He was doing God's work, but for them it would be their work and not the work of the Father. Bottom line, they missed the miracle!

Chapter 6
Maniacs -The Certifiable

Luke 4:33-37 gives an account of Jesus dealing with a person with behavioral problems just like in modern day society, handling snakes I like to call it. Because people with behavioral problems were dealt with by Jesus in a particular way. See, it's the snake in the person causing the behavior. Why look at it like this?

Well, it's not like snake charming, but subdueing these pesky animals who crawl through our lives, slithering their way into our affairs and creating havoc in men. Yes, it's demons that **inhabit** people that are the snakes in our lives that we don't see coming or we would move away to protect ourselves. They subtly slide into our lives and before you know it, you're starring one right in the face, too close to escape, so you freeze not knowing what to do. Sssssssssssssss!

But Jesus was good at handling them. I would guess that 40 days and nights dealing with them in the wilderness (during his fast) has got to give you skills!

Nope, he didn't just contend with them the last day of the fast, but every day, every hour, hour after hour…. FOR FORTY DAYS, I believe cause I've never know a snake, or demon for that matter to cut anybody some slack. If you don't believe me, start fasting for three days and let me know how many times you wrestle with thoughts to eat, or give up, or whimp out and only God knows (and now you), what else you will be attacked with to get off your square (your commitment to serve the Lord and subdue your appetites).

You have to get to know your enemy pretty well by then. So in this scripture he shows us how to deal with them, QUICKLY. He grabs it by the proverbial tail, like he told Moses to do, and executes their demise. Verse 34 states:

"And in the synagogue there was a man possessed by a demon, an evil (or unclean) spirit, began shouting at Jesus, "Go away! Why are you interfering with us, Jesus of Nazareth? Have you come to destroy us? I know who you are,

the Holy One of God!" Jesus cut him short. "Be quiet! Come out of the man." He ordered. At that, the demon threw the man to the floor as the crowd watched; then it came out of him without hurting him further.

Luke 4:33-35

I can't help but picture a bully who's time is up. He gets angry at having to leave his victim or his "scene" so he throws something (the man in this case) or has his "fit." This goes to show how he despises those who know how to deal with him and defeat him effectively, it an intimidation gesture. I know those of you that are parents have seen this behavior in your younger children (and maybe some of your teens too) so you know what it looks like! So Jesus shows us an important technique in snake wrestling, quickly and directly by saying "Be quiet!" then he commands, "Come out of the man!" Instantly he is cut down, just as even the demon himself predicts he could be destroyed. And because of Jesus' authority and who that demon knows he is (the Holy One of God), he preceives that if commanded, he will have to get up from this territory. Yes, in God's health care system, we don't counsel demons, we cast them out.

Note the response of the crowd, since the demon's public response effected them as they looked on:

"Amazed, the people exclaimed, "What authority and power this man's words possess. Even evil spirits obey him, and they flee at his command!" The news about Jesus spread through every village in the entire region."

Luke 4: 36-37

Now the crowd sees how to deal with the snake, using authority and speaking (words) with confidence (faith). And I'm sure they were happy about what Jesus did, who wants that bully (demon) living in their community!

In God's Health Care System, He knows the cures. The cure to some behavioral problems and mental illnesses according to God is dealing with the demons. Even the first lesson God showed Moses to demonstrating His power was how to handle a snake (symbolic of demonic forces) by taking his staff and turning it into one and then he uses this knowledge to deal with Pharoah

(Exodus 4:2-5).

The Many

"That evening many demon-possessed people were brought to Jesus. He cast out the evil spirits with a simple command, and he healed all the sick." Matthew 8:16-17

Jesus again uses his words (authority by speaking) to cast out demonic spirits for people to receive healing. Note that this technique I have never seen in all my 30 years of practice to cure someone. In other words, you will only see this procedure in the God's Health Care System And note also that demons do exist and cause many of our mental health and behavioral problems.

Ever wonder why you can go to the hospital with a problem and the doctors run all those tests, and they come back negative and it makes you feel like your going crazy because you know you're sick and in pain. You can't run a test and the result come back "there's three demons in there". And even if there was, what they gonna do about it?? Cast it out?? Then bill you for that?? (I can't keep a straight face while I type this). Nope. Your're, well.......out of luck. They don't even suggest you get that dealt with on Sunday or the Sabbath as the Pharisees in the bible protested Jesus healing people on that day. Yes, deliverance services will not be held in your hospital room or doctor's office, even in a faith based hospital.

Legion

And then there was the man, the maniac of the Gadarenes:

"So they arrived at the
other side of the lake, in the
region of the Garasenes. When
Jesus climbed out of the boat, a
man possessed by an evil spirit
came out from the tombs to
meet him. This man lived in the
burial caves and could no longer
be restrained, even with a chain.
Whenever he was put into chains
and shackles, as he often was, he
snapped the chains from his
wrists and smashed the shackles.
No one was strong enough to
subdue him. Day and night he
wandered among the burial
caves and in the hills, howling

and cutting himself with sharp stones.

When Jesus was still some distance away, the man saw him, ran to meet him, and bowed low before him. With a shriek, he screamed, "Why are you interfering with me, Jesus, Son of the Most High God? In the name of God, I beg you, don't torture me!" For Jesus had already said to the spirit." Come out of the man, you evil spirit."

Then Jesus demanded, "What is your name?" And he replied, "My name is Legion, because there are many of us inside this man." Then the evil spirits begged him again and again not to send them to some distant place.

There happened to be a large herd of pigs feeding on the hillside nearby. "Send us into those pigs, " the spirits begged. "Let us enter them."

So Jesus gave them permission. The evil spirits came out of the man and entered the pigs, and the entire herd of about 2,000 pigs plunged down the steep hillside into the lake and drowned in the water.

The herdsmen fled to the nearby town and the

surrounding countryside,
spreading the news as they ran.
People rushed out to see what
had happened. A crowd soon
gathered around Jesus, and they
saw the man who had been
possessed by the legion of
demons. He was sitting there
fully clothed and perfectly sane,
and they were all afraid. Then
those who had seen what
happened told the others about
the demon-possed man and the
pigs. And the crowd began
pleading with Jesus to go away
and leave them alone.

As Jesus was getting into
the boat, the man who had been

demon possessed begged to go with him. But Jesus said, "No, go home to your family, and tell them everything the Lord has done for you and how merciful he has been." So the man started off to visit the Ten Towns of that region and began to proclaim the great things Jesus had done for him and everyone was amazed at what he told them.

Mark 5:1-20 (NLT)

This is one of the worse cases of demonically possessed people recorded in the bible. A demoniac is a person whose personality has been invaded by one or more demons, who at will can speak and act through their human victim, deranging both his mind and body.

In this condition, he had the outward appearance of severe mental illness with isolation by living in caves and burial grounds, defying restraints (normally causing a person to get an emergency injected sedative or anti anxiety agent in a hospital today), super human strength, and howling. This man was cutting himself, which is a common symptom seen in teenagers with mental health issues today along with piercing, tatooing and embedding foreign objects.

In the earth cursed system of health, mental illness is not generally treated successfully because it does not deal with the root of the problems as Jesus shows us repeatedly in the gospels. Funding for mental health clinics and mental health care facilites or centers have drastically decreased over the years. So treating mental health is getting harder. You will find most people are given medications that do not cure their problems and the psychiatric field in general have problems with diagnosing, prescribing and getting people to cooperate with treatment modalities. This is one medical field that is dominated by pharmacutical intervention and many are over, under and inappropriately medicated. Some psychiatric conditions can be cured with just better nutrition that promotes and supports healthy brain function.

But Jesus cast out many demons which manifested in behavioral and physical problems or epileptic seizures that plagued and tormented people.

I couldn't help but wonder how the maniac of Gadara could develop such a serious and chronic condition to this extreme, 2000 demons (demonic infestation I like to call it)! Then I remembered where Jesus noted how this happends in a later discussion with the nay sayers regarding his authority to cast out demons saying that:

"When an evil spirit leaves a person, it goes into the desert, searching for rest. But when it finds none, it says, 'I will return to the person I came from.' So it returns and finds that its former home is all swept and in order.

Luke 11:24-26

If this be examined, it could explain how a person who manages to get well could have 1 demon leave, that brings 7 demons back with him, (that's 8 total) to inhabit him if he fails. He could suffer from 2000 demons after some 250 attempts to get better (250 divided by 8)! That means over a 20 year period he could try 12 times a year!

This is also why the demons begged Jesus to let them go into the pigs; otherwise they would have roamed around with nowhere to inhabit and "not find rest". They can't do any damage without a host. Even so, look what they did to those pigs! I also understand that pigs were used as sacrifices to the idols of that region, so allowing the legion to go into the pigs and they plundge down the hillside into the lake was Jesus way of shutting down the idol worship there.

I personally cannot believe this man did not try to get help over the years, since the scripture states that others had attempted to restrain him and especially because of the way he came out to meet Jesus when he arrived on the shore (bowed down and worshipped him). Yes, he got help in general, even if it were from the wrong health care system. There had to be some part of him that desired relief to do that. But external cleaning up without true regeneration invites Satan to return with seven viler spirits. Only Jesus could really help him, and you.

Chapter 7

Just Because I Love YOU

*"Soon afterward Jesus
went with his disciples to the
village of Nain, and a large
crowd followed him. A funeral
procession was coming out as he
approached the village gate.
The young man who had died
was a widow's only son, and a
large crowd from the village was
with her. When the Lord saw
her, his heart overflowed with
compassion. "Don't cry!" he
said. Then he walked over to the
coffin and touched it, and the*

*bearers stopped. "Young man,"
he said, "I tell you get up." Then
the dead boy sat up and began
to talk! And Jesus gave him back
to his mother. Great fear swept
the crowd, and they praised God,
saying, "A mighty prophet has
risen among us: and God has
visited his people today." And
the news about Jesus spread
throughout Judea and the
surrounding countryside.*

Luke 7:11-19 (NLT)

Jesus walking through this town comes to what we know today is an event that would stop our normal daily activities. Funerals have always been

something that people have to
stop what they are normally
doing to "attend to". It causes
us to stop our lives to grieve and
be sorrowful. We can't even
continue our lives the way they
were before because now this
person's absence will change our
lives forever. Now we have to
rearrange our lives and forever
be aware that some one is now
missing and this hole is felt. I
have never liked the reality of
death. As a child, I always
wondered why do we have to
tolerate this event, this problem-
-dying. Why do we ever have to
have "death" in the picture of

life. Who invented this phenomenon? What do you mean, they won't ever come back. That's cruel! These were the questions I asked as a young person. No one is happy about it but rather we sit in shock if it is a sudden death or weary if it has been someone dying slowly. We sit in fear really wondering who will be next or when it will happen to us. We can never prepare enough for it. But take a look at God's perspective.

<u>The Widow</u>

The woman in this scripture is stated to be a widow, a woman who has already

suffered the death of a loved
one and it's grief, her spouse,
and now facing parenting alone.
Only to be put in the situation
again with her son dying and
leaving her completely alone,
probably without any financial
help since widows in this day
were a chief concern of the
spiritual community in terms of
giving along with those who
were poor.

I wonder why her son
died? Sickness or disease or
generational family problem or
maybe a tragic event? I guess
this is why there was such a
crowd with her, something that

would not only have her in turmoil but the whole community was effected and came out to give their support and presence. Jesus seeing all this was overflowing with compassion. He had a reputation for help and supporting women so he stopped to become an influencial part of what was happening. He was not asked but responded because God wants to solve our problems and be an active part of our lives. He approaches the situation and tells the woman not to weep saying to her, "don't cry", not to

console her but to encourage
her because he wants to solve
her problems. God wants to
stop the procession in your life
(of tragedy and problems), heal
your body, rearrange the events
of your life and get the glory for
it. "Beauty for Ashes" as they
say. No one else can perform a
miracle in your life, **change** your
life forever, resurrect something
that has died in your life. Yes,
He can speak to us when we are
dead and gone (in our situations)
and tell us to arise from our
situations, downfalls or
misfortunes. His ultimate
concern is that we live a useful

life in this world and are prepared to live with Him in the next world. In His health care system, there is no such thing as too late. Especially, since God is a god of second chances and especially if he gives those second chances so that we can get it right this time. Could he have raised her son from the dead for a second chance to make a decision for eternal life, to get it right this time? This is not the motive of the earth cursed system of health. In the earth cursed health care system, they resuscitate people and bring them back to life in this world, but God resurrected people to bring them back so they can have life in the eternal world also.

Chapter 8

Faith Awards

The Centurion

This section is an interesting story about a man who is a Roman centurion (Luke 7:1-10) or officer who lived amoung the Jewish people and loved them. Yes, you heard me, a Roman who had an anti-Roman attitude toward the people he had to be in charge over. So much so that he built a worship center for them. When his "highly valued slave" (who I'm sure wasn't Roman) became seriously ill, he asked some of the Jewish leaders to beg Jesus to come and heal him. They even told Jesus that this Roman was not your average Roman in that he even built them a synagogue, so he should be treated "like us."

When the officer started to think about what he had requested and the fact that he was asking the one he believed was "the Messiah" to come to his home, he backed out in humility. He didn't even feel worthy for him to come there, yet alone met him in person. He just unselfishly wanted to help stop his servant suffering an imminent death. It was a long shot but he was willing to try. So he sends a second somewhat unusual message back through his friends. This time to say "on second thought don't bother to come because I'm ashamed of who I am and the things I've done (as a Roman). In my culture as a commanding officer and one under command if you just speak it, it will be done. You have authority and power to get things done so just say it and my servant will be helped."

Jesus, shocked at the second request, knows that this was a man who came to God for help that understood the concept of Jesus' authority and what the kingdom has to offer and he even knew how to get it, BY FAITH. Well, by the time his friends got back, his servant was healed. Jesus says to the crowd that here is A ROMAN who has more faith than the whole Jewish nation. What a man!

Isn't it nice to know that you're doing the right thing, at the right time, for the right reasons. No doctor needed, or health assessment done, just an understanding of the kingdom and it's use of power and authority. No side effects or

complications either. This is a
critical concept in God's Health
Care System and the kingdom
that must be understood that is
a game changer. So the servant
is healed, a reward of faith.

The Paralyzed Man

In Luke 5:17 Jesus is back
home and gets his roof torn off
because a group of men believe
Jesus can heal their friend or
relative. But just before this is
mentioned, it states that there
were Pharisees and doctors of
the law sitting by, which were
come out of every town of

Galilee, and Judaea, and Jerusalem: **"and that the Power of the Lord was present to heal them" the scripture says.** Yes, "power" to heal even the hypocrites and skeptics who came to criticize the health care system, and the man.

And another thing is mentioned, that Jesus was there teaching the people. Meaning the teaching about the Kingdom and its health care system was facilitating this power being present. This generated the people's faith to be stirred up by hearing what can be done.

So, Jesus is brought a man, on a bed, with "palsy" medically know has paralysis. After they can't get him to Jesus because of the crowd, they go through the roof because they know he can heal him. Remember, when an act of faith is presented, you qualify for a miracle.

But Jesus says something unexpected. "Your sins are forgiven." I never heard sin being addressed in the clinical setting (which is a first priority with God I might add, part of His history and physical), because they do not address your spiritual state or your totality.

But God knows that is the one thing that separates us from his kingdom. This fact Jesus immediately brings to light. When you come to Jesus, the first thing he asks us to do is confess our sins, then you get forgiveness. In other words, first things first. But now that your sins are forgiven, you are a child of God with the rights and privileges of the Kingdom of God! Then what do you deserve as God's child? Your inheritance! That's right, healing…. the children's bread. And it's free to you because Jesus will pay for you. That's why you'll never go broke or bankrupt from using God's Health Care System. He paid the price on the cross for us all.

However, Jesus' fame had gone out into the region and his activities are now being monitored by the religious community leaders (to get ammunition against him for his dismissal so to speak). They murmured about Jesus response, but he asked them which thing is easier to do, forgive this man's sins or heal him? So then with a demonstration of his authority, from God, he tells the man to "rise take up your bed and go home". So, he jumps up and goes home, rejoicing. Yes, take up your bed of troubles and go home (to show your family you're healed). Jesus healed that man to demonstrate who he really is to all who believe. He's the man that comes on the scene with a message and a health care system. Now the people must make a decision about what is happening here because they are confronted with evidence, a very powerful and persuasive proof that He could be the Messiah.

Chapter 9

Ask

Jesus Heals a Man with Leprosy

"In one of the villages, Jesus met a man with an advanced case of leprosy. When the man saw Jesus, he bowed with his face to the ground begging to be healed. "Lord," he said, "if you are willing, you can heal me and make me clean."

Jesus reached out and touched him. "I am willing," he said. "Be healed!" And instantly the leprosy disappeared. Then

Jesus instructed him not to tell anyone what had happened. He said, "Go to the priest and let him examine you. Take along the offering required in the Law of Moses for those who have been healed of leprosy. This will be a public testimony that you have been cleansed."   Luke 5 12-14

Here Jesus meets a man, who from the earth cursed system perspective is now at the end of his disease condition with a chronic or an advanced stage of leprosy. At this time in history, there was no antibiotics that could be used as there are today. So, this man had to beg Jesus to heal him if he was to survive this crippling disease (disfiguring skin lesions, and peripheral nerve damage due to mycobacterium leper bacteria). Today sufferer's need only take multidrug therapy for a year with antibiotics to cure leprosy. But back then this man had to take the initiative, as we should do, and asked Jesus to cure him. He makes a statement saying he knows Jesus can heal him, words expressing his faith. But he also says something I think we should acknowledge, and that is that God can make us clean or holy.

Yep, it his will for us to be in righteous standing, sanctified (cleansed from all diseases) by his power.

Again, it is important to know that in God's Health Care System, as he states in this story, it is His will for you to be clean from an infirmity. He says to "be ye holy as I am holy". So, he tells the man he is willing to help him and instantly heals him with a *touch* and his *words of authority* and again in Mark 1:41 being moved with compassion. He then tells him how he wants him to respond to his miracle, to follow spiritual procedure by giving his offering to God and to give his "testimony" that God has cleansed him. This way others will be shown that God wants us to have healing or tell others what he is willing to do for us. He even tells him to show his gratitude by giving the appropriate offering. And notice he got his healing just because he asked. Not because of our performance or our status or education. No nah, he won't do that for me responses. It's because he cares about what happens to us or how he can make our lives better. So,

where's the no, I don't want you
healed!

Chapter 10
Oh, I See!

There were several people in the bible who experience healing in the area of the 6 senses. Some couldn't hear but there were those who were blind that Jesus healed in unusual ways. Three of them I would like to mention because your faith is at stake and I want you to know that if you agree, nothing is impossible.

In John 9:1-41, a blind man gets sight. It is the sixth miraculous healing noted in the gospels. This is an illustration of light and illumination for the new life to be found in Christ and the Kingdom of God. This is what happened:

"As Jesus was walking along, he saw a man who had been blind from birth. "Rabbi," his disciples asked him, "why was this man born blind? Was it because of his own sins or his parents' sins?'

"It was not because of his sins or his parents' sins, " **Jesus answered.** "This happened so the power of God could be seen in him. We must quickly carry out the tasks assigned us by the

Then he spit on the ground, made mud with the saliva, and spread the mud over the blind man's eyes. He told him, *So the man went and washed and came back seeing!"*

John 9:1-41 (NLT)

Now I'm guessing that your reaction to this is probably what mine was, "what a strange thing

to do to get someone healed."
But I consider some of the things
modern medicine does to cure
people of their ailments can't
begin to compare. I honestly
think cutting off body parts or
joint replacements are pretty
extreme in view of the fact that
the human body is made with
divine intelligence (the God
engineered ability to be it's own
physician) and is well able to
heal itself of it's problems if you
give it the 90 essential nutrients
daily that it needs and don't
abuse it with toxic chemicals,
diets and and harsh life styles. In
other words, it knows how to fix

itself without guessing. After all, that's how our viruses are cured. They don't have meds for them, yet the human body can defeat them or everybody would have viruses. Our immune system is designed to fight infections and invaders if you give it what it needs. It is your greatest defense against diseases. In tandum with the liver, which eliminates toxins, you have a powerful front against most everything. But, what do you think?

His neighbors and others who knew him as a blind beggar asked each other, "Isn't this the man who used to sit and beg?"

Some said he was, and others said, "No, he just looks like him!" But the beggar kept saying, "Yes, I am the same one!"

They asked, "Who healed you? What happened?" He told them, "The man they call Jesus made mud and spread it over my eyes and told me, 'Go to the pool of Siloan and wash yourself.' So I went and washed, and now I can see!" "Where is he now?" they asked. "I don't know, " he replied.

Then they took the man who had been blind to the Pharisees, because it was on the Sabbath (I have already discussed this issue in the chapter called "Holidays") that Jesus had made mud and healed him. The Pharisees asked the man all about it. So he told them, "He put the mud over my eyes, and when I washed it away, I could see!"

Some of the Pharisees said, "This man Jesus is not from God for he is working on the Sabbath."

It amazed me here that they completely ignored the miracle to note that it had been done ON THE SABBATH. Dah!

"Others said, "But how could an ordinary sinner do such miraculous signs?" So there was a deep division of opinion among them."

This is when I think they are finally getting to the most serious question about this incident and God's Health Care System in general. When you are healed by God, it is the miraculous. Yes, you don't get this kind of healing from the world's earth cursed system. And this is why you should not rely on getting this kind of result from it. You will not get this gift anywhere other than from God.

And he wants you to know that. Later, you will see why so stay with me on this discourse. And call him what you may (a sinner) but even Jesus said:

"But if I do his work (that of the Heavenly Father), believe in the evidence of the miraculous works I have done, even if you don't believe me. Then you will know and understand that the Father is in me, and I am in the Father."
John 10:38

This lack of belief in God's results in His Health Care System brought a deep division among the people and it still does the same today. People have a hard time understanding that it is possible to receive healing like this. Look at how the religious community responded to a man who represented the evidence or proof that the power of God works.

"Then the Pharisees again questioned the man who had been blind and demanded, "What's your opinion about this man who healed you?"

The man replied, "I think he must be a prophet."

The Jewish leaders still refused to believe the man had

been blind and could now see, so they called in his parents. They asked them, "Is this your son? Was he born blind? If so, how can he now see?"

His parents replied, "We know this is our son and that he was born blind, but we don't know how he can see or who healed him. Ask him. He is old enough to speak for himself." His parents said this because they were afraid of the Jewish leaders, who had announced that anyone saying Jesus was the Messiah would be expelled from the synagogue. That's why he said, "He is old enough. Ask him."

This is why I believe the medical system will not come clean about their inability to truly help people in today's world, especially America's system of health. If they were to admit the fact that people get worse in their care, all would turn away and look for another solution and their credibility would be gone forever. Most people who do find out, find out too late or die before they do.

Our health care system is one of reductionistic (good for trauma, surgery when really needed and a hand full of infections) medicine (also know as allopathic medicine) and not wholistic (herbalisy, chiropractors, acupucture, chinese, ayurvedic) or naturopathic medicine. The difference is they are not trained in the proper therapeutics to cure chronic illness. But they have monopolized health care and put themselves in first place and practically made it legal for no one else to help you. They only know what they have been trained for and it is a very small piece of the medical pie in the world. Unfortunately, they are prideful and this medicine in our country is the leading cause of bankruptcy and death in the United States. I discuss this in my book **Perfect Cures for Perfect Health** (http://amzn.to/2Dz23a0).

"So for the second time they called in the man who had been blind and told him, "God should get the glory for this, because we know this man Jesus is a sinner."

"I don't know whether he is a sinner, " the man replied. "But I know this: I was blind, and now I can see!"

But what did he do?" they asked. "How did he heal you?"

"Look!" the man exclaimed. "I told you once. Didn't you listen? Why do you want to hear it again? Do you want to become his disciples, too?"

Then they cursed him and said, "You are his disciple, but we are disciples of Moses! We know God spoke to Moses, but we don't even know where this man comes from."

"Why, that's very strange!" the man replied. "He healed my eyes, and yet you don't know *where he comes from? We know that God doesn't listen to sinners, but he is ready to hear those who worship him and do his will. Ever since the world began, no one has been able to open the eyes of someone born blind. If this man were not from God, he couldn't have done it."*

"You were born a total sinner!" they answered. "Are you trying to teach us?" And they threw him out of the synagogue."

One of the reasons that Jesus used this as a method of healing (using his spit and mixing it with mud) is because it is symbolic of how the things of God are detestible to the unbeliever. The gospel or anything of the God Kingdom to man is detestible and offending. Then going to wash it off as, yes you guessed it, an act of faith, the part we have to play in our God's Health Care System. Most people respond to God by rejection because these two systems or kingdoms are diametrically opposed to one another. Listen to the end of the matter:

Spiritual Blindness

When Jesus heard what had happened, he found the man

and asked, "Do you believe in the Son of Man?"

The Man answered, "Who is he, sir? I want to believe in him." "You have seen him," **Jesus said,** "and he is speaking to you!"

"Yes, Lord, I believe!" the man said. And he worshiped Jesus.

Then Jesus told him, "I entered this world to render judgment--to give sight to the blind and to show those who think they see that they are blind."

Some Pharisees who were standing nearby heard him and asked, "Are you saying we're blind?"

If you were blind, you wouldn't be guilty," **Jesus replied.**

"But you remain guilty because you claim you can see.

John 9:1-41

Remember I mentioned that you would see why you should not rely on this system of health for your healing. I have listed some exceptions but generally it can not be relied upon because they can not see because of their spiritual blindness. They don't know that they don't know.

There was a second man from Bethesda who Jesus used spit as a method to bring about his healing from blindness listed in Mark 8:22-26 but he leads him by the hand completely outside the village before he does this.

One important aspect in God's Health Care System and his Kingdom is the fact that we have to trust Him to use it. Have you ever been lead around blindfolded in a childhood game or otherwise? How did it feel? It may have been a genuine time where you had to put your trust in another. Here, the man from Bethesda had to put his trust in Jesus leading him around, then allowing him to put spit on his eye before he could receive his sight. Have I mention in the previous healing, to be spit on is either an humiliating experience or in this case, a humbling experience. But the question is what are you willing to do to be a part of God's Kingdom and His desire for you to have divine health? What will you do to get healing? Are you willing to use unconventional methods to receive health (root word here in health is heal). It is no different today than it was in bible times because what is happening today has not changed from then to now.

In fact, we tend to trust in all the technology that fascinate us and modern procedures that astound us because of the culture. We forget they have disadvantages. Then we don't assess their consequences BEFORE we use them. We don't count the real cost. In God's Kingdom, he "adds no sorrow to it" referring to his blessings the Bible states. There will be no negative consequences. As a matter of fact, God's blessings are sooo awesome that he had to warn us, as well as the children of Israel to not forsake him once we receive them. Blessings are more dangerous than misfortune because they cause us to drift away from God in our happiness and fullfillment.

I recently came across a testimony about a man who's wife was suffering from a vision problem. He is a marine. They were told that an increase in the strength of her glasses would help, but it didn't. Then the doctor finally told her that her retina scan showed an aggressive form of macula degenration, a serious eye disease that destroys your central eye vision. They gave her 6 months before she would be completely blind.

So he researched all types of interventions for eye cures, but none were appealing, affordable or safe. When one day this marine found information on their computer about how to commit suicide that his wife had been looking up, he decided to turn to God for help and prayed.

In the middle of things getting progressively worse, he got a call to be deployed for a training exercise in the Australian outback where they would be teaming up with the soldiers there for survelience missions looking for drug smugglers, human trafficing, assimlum seekers and illegal foreign vessels.

On the third day, they were learning techniques from a soldier there and he suddenly saw a boat out on the water. When he and his team looked out on the water they didn't see any boat. But the soldier insisted it was there. They took their binocular and look out on the horizon and low and behold there was a boat there that they could barely see, EVEN WITH THE BINOCULARS. When they radio contacted his unit they intercepted 4 men who were smuggling 2000 lbs of drugs with an estimated value of $14 million.

When the marine talked to the soldier later he asked him how could he see that vessel out there like that. He left and came back with a paper and pen and wrote down the secret to his extraordinary vision. It was a list of foods that are indigious to their culture that for generations had given his people "super sight". This phenomanon has been documented by studies from the local university in their area which reveals his people's vision to be 4 times better. In fact, his people have the best vision on the globe. He never saw that man again.

Needless to say, the marine took this information home and with the help of a medical researcher they adapted this information for use in America and have done studies on how well it works and why. His wife was the first to use it and in 21 days her sight was restored to 20/20 vision. 93% of the people on the study also received 20/20 vision. Now some 51,297 people have benefited from the protocol! I put his information at the end of this book.

Was this deployment a coincidence? Does God want to solve your health problems? I believe when you turn to Him, he will help you. Even if he has to send you half way around the world to do it! I found his testimony just days before the publishing of this book.

So what do you want to do about God, His Health Care System and the health that is

available to you? Where will you
go from here?

Prayer of Salvation

If you have not made a decision to become a citizen of the Kingdom of God, Jesus is the door, or the way, the truth and the life. Here is a simple prayer you can say to receive the gift (of salvation) that keeps on giving:

"Dear God, I want to be a part of your family. You said in Your Word that if I acknowledge that you raised Jesus from the dead, and that I accept Him as my Lord and Savior, I would be saved. So God, I now say that I believe You raised Jesus from the dead and that He is alive and well. I accept Him now as my personal Lord and Savior. I accept my salvation from sin right now.

I am now saved. Jesus is my Lord. Jesus is my Savior. Thank you, Father God, for forgiving me, saving me, and giving me eternal life with You. Amen!"

WELCOME TO THE KINGDOM OF GOD!

Please go to a bible believing church to be taught about the Kingdom and to learn the Word of God. It will transform your life.

After you read this book if you feel like I've provided you with quality content and valuable information, would you do me a HUGE favor please? I would appreciate it if you would write me a great five-star customer review for this book on Amazon. Hopefully our paths will cross at some point in our lives and we can meet each other in person. I pray that you will be blessed with perfect health, abundant wealth and never-ending happiness! Feel free to contact me at the email address below. God bless you!

Shellyjenkins13@gmail.com

The website for the healing mention in chapter 10 on sight is:

(www.outbackvisionprotocol.com)

5. Aaron's Preschool Book For 3
Year Olds: A Little Boy's
Adventures

http://amzn.to/2qzFgo5

6. Aaron and Aniya's Beginners
Bible, A Children's First bible
Book

http://amzn.to/2t5vCau

About the Author

Shelly Jenkins is a native of Chicago, Illinois and has been a believer in Christ since young adulthood. An avid bible scholar, certified natural health teacher, bachelors prepared registered nurse for more than 32 years, she has worked in a variety of nursing areas including Maternal Child Health, Nursing Education, and Child Welfare Services. Currently a school nurse for over 12 years and legal nurse consultant, she has a passion for health, healing and wellness through a biblical perspective.

An artist in her spare time, she is a mother of two and a grandmother of four and is currently living in Columbus, Ohio.

Shelly Jenkins

Email:

shellyjenkins13@gmail.com

Website:

www.godshealthcaresystem.com

www.ingramcontent.com/pod-product-compliance
Lightning Source LLC
Chambersburg PA
CBHW070659250726
48662CB00001B/205